I0476504

Prologue

I wrote the first edition of this little book as a way to answer the ongoing question—where can I find healthcare data? I had my resources arranged by bookmarks, links, and notes on pages. Not easy to find when I was busily writing about health economics, disease state awareness, or research articles.

I quickly published this little book and continue to be surprised by its popularity and utility. This past year was a busy one for data. National Health Statistics conference, NIH meetings, even a trip to the White House Conference on Aging introduced new sources of data—and Tableau Data Visualization conference created opportunity to explore the data, reinforce my skills, and better communicate using an important tool for creating our narratives—graphical representation.

My goal is to create value at a price point easily accessible to everyone. It is written, "edited", and published by yours truly so typos are my own.

I am going to review and freshen early pages and add a section on a few more data sources. If you find value here please write a review. When I know what you value, I can share useful tools—and you don't need to travel!

Introduction

Here is the opportunity as I see it. Innovative advances in medicine and healthcare delivery are being made each and every day. The patient-level delivery of care is the real determinant of an intervention. So while technology innovation is important, what we really need is process innovation. We need to deliver the right care to the right people in the right time frame and right sequence.

The EHR/EMR system is being integrated into daily practice on an escalating basis and to achieve the vision promised by information technology—we need collaborative efforts. Financial costs continue to be aggregated and analyzed at the specialty or service department level. What we need to do is focus on the costs of treating patients over their full cycle of care. Let's stop measuring the wrong things the wrong way...

Data is everywhere and it seems that everyone has a

handle on this new source of useable information—
but do they? In healthcare especially much of the
data is behind a firewall, proprietary and/or access is
monetized as part of a business model or opportunity.

Perhaps there are glimpses here and there visible at
conferences or embedded in news articles but what
do you do with your own data?

Unless you have deep pockets and can afford industry
data access, it isn't likely you are going to spend
thousands and thousands of dollars to access **IMS
data,** a leader in the billion-dollar pharmaceutical
data industry. I observed my bookshelf and although I
have quite a few books about healthcare data, I rely
on only a chapter here and there from each book.

The idea for short chapter books specific to a
business need was generated. I curated the most
frequent questions from my blog at
www.dataanddonuts.org and created a publication
strategy for short topics as an introduction and a

quick how-to resource.

This format is also easily updated and can be integrated into a curated series based on your own level and interests.

Let's see where we can find some useful data for our proposals, websites, corporate blogs, brand content, and digital communication strategies.

Patient Level Data

There are a variety of sources of longitudinal patient data (LPD). The data is de-identified and can be collected from health claims data, pharmacy records, electronic medical records, and any other source that tracks data linearly over a period of time.

What type of information can you potentially derive from patient level data?

Prevalence and incidence, demographics, treatment protocols, patient referrals, prescriptions, days on treatment, sequence of drug regimens, screening, vaccinations, adherence, are just a few examples of the type of data available. I have extensive experience analyzing electronic medical record data useful for measuring how specific drugs are being prescribed and by whom, what are the dosages, how have prescribing trends shifted over time (are they influenced by sampling for example), what percentage of patient population is comorbid, treatment sequence data--the granularity of new, switch, add-on, etc. dynamics are also relevant. Why are patients switching? What are the outcomes on the new regimens?

The value of including this type of data in content documents or reporting is to measure actual prescribing and patient management data in real time. Patient-level data removes the bias inherent in survey instruments and allows deeper dives into the data. For example, you can evaluate data by indication, line of treatment, market dynamics, and comorbidity.

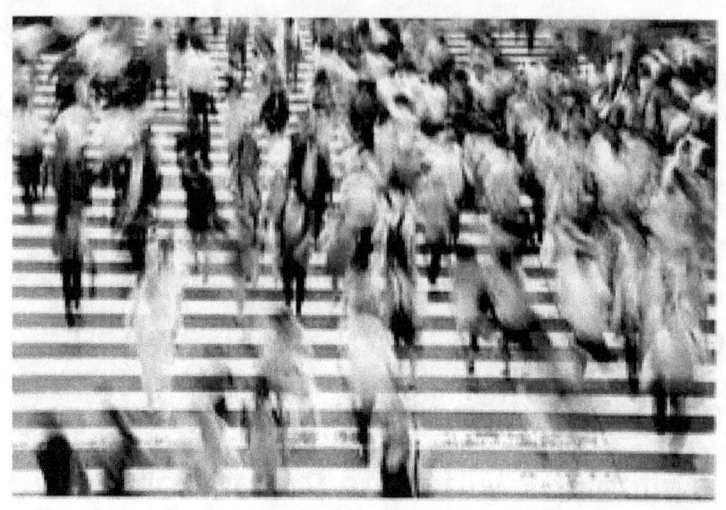

Industry stakeholders are making claims of value and requesting that brand strategies, continuing educational programs, and digital media advertising integrate a narrative voice. The ability to identify where data might be relevant throughout a product or brand lifecycle can be an effective strategy to engage an audience and facilitate relevant discussion.

Patient data collected over time in a linear manner provides insights during all phases of a product lifecycle. Integrated into a needs assessment to contextualize a perceived gap in clinical care or to determine efficacy or evaluation of market strengths and/or weaknesses collected prior to launch establish the landscape to identify facilitators or barriers to uptake.

In addition, the ability to stratify data by cohorts may be useful in identifying clinical trial participants, create meaningful endpoints, and create a value proposition.

Assets moving into phase III benefit from positioning data relevant for pricing strategies and value statement refinement prior to commercialization and identification for targeting, messaging, and promotion.

Research and Development (R&D) launch is no longer the end-post. Market access is optimized by observational studies demonstrating real world evidence and multiple sources of data are needed to continuously adjust value messaging in the shifting landscape of new and emergent therapies. Additional data is needed as patents expire and generic formulations require efficacy and safety messages.

Data of interest to industry and physicians

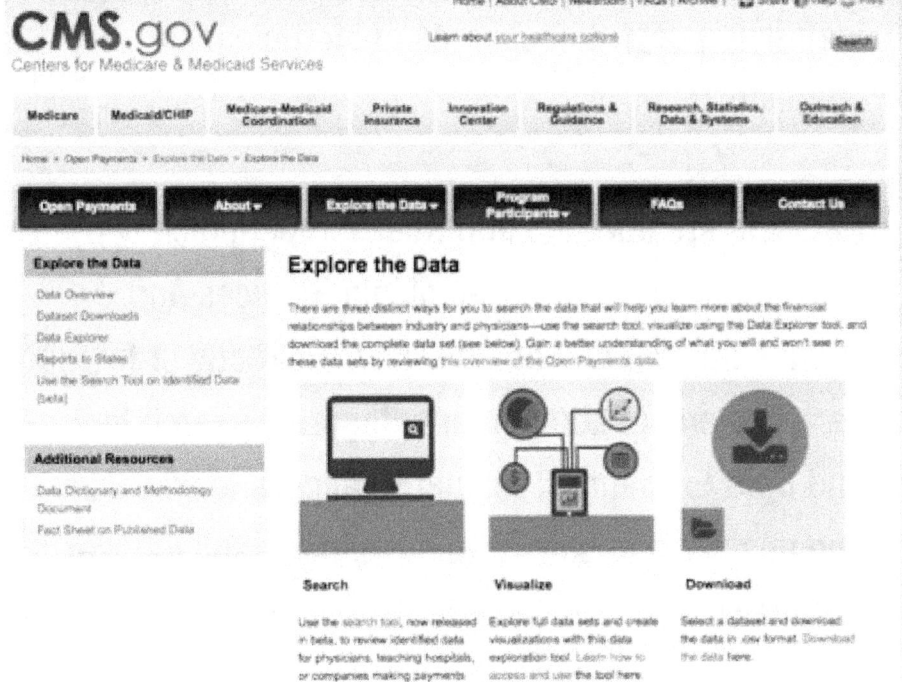

https://www.cms.gov/OpenPayments/Explore-the-Data/Explore-the-Data.html

There have been influential posts in social media successful at creating awareness around abusive trends in Medicare payments to providers. The source of the data has been in part the transparency required by provisions in the Affordable Care Act. The ability to drill into reimbursement data at the regional, provider, and therapeutic level is instrumental in identifying potential sources of inefficiencies and spiraling costs.

Datasets are updated and released periodically by Centers for Medicare & Medicaid Services and include payments made directly, indirectly or by third party payers. In addition an integrated search tool and Data Exchange Tool allows access to visualize and analyze datasets or to download a full dataset. The views available include **data lens**, datasets, charts, maps, calendars, filtered views, external datasets, forms, and even APIs.

"With Data Lens, governments can finally shift from simple, data-centric citizen interaction to an information-centric experience. Government data becomes dramatically more accessible and impactful for citizens, community advocates, journalists, and employees."

Data of Interest for Providers and Consumers

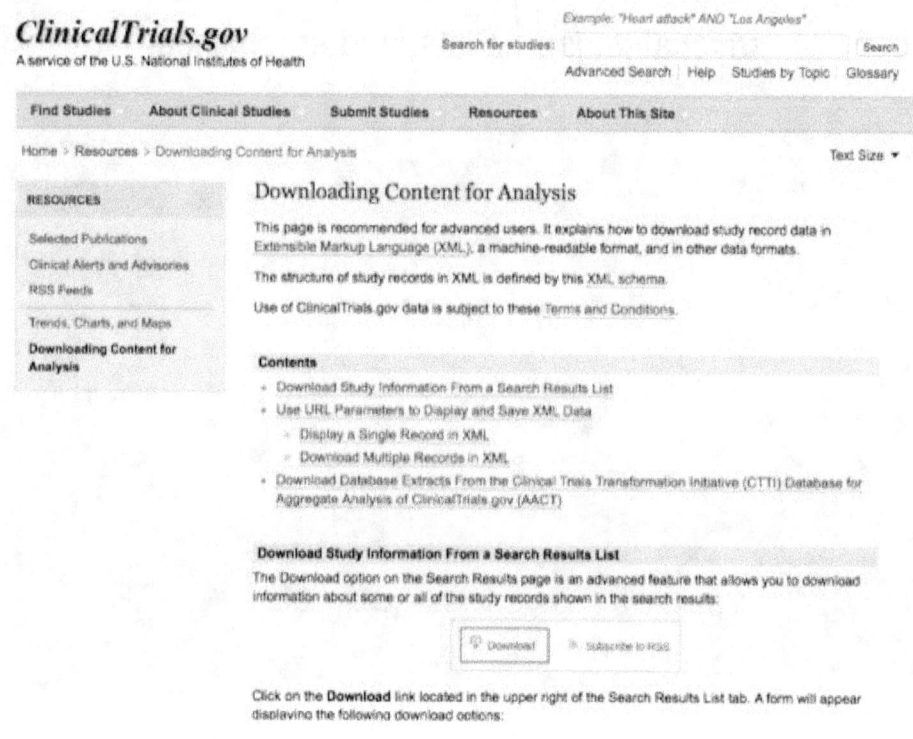

https://clinicaltrial.gov/ct2/resources/download

Clinicaltrial.gov is a useful "web-based resource that provides patients, their family members, health care professionals, researchers, and the public with easy access to information on publicly and privately supported clinical studies on a wide range of diseases and conditions".

The National Library of Medicine (NLM) at the National Institutes of Health (NIH includes information that is updated by the sponsor or principal investigator of the clinical study. At specific points during the longitudinal timeline or often submitted after the study ends data is uploaded to the site. This database of clinical studies is a "registry" and "results database."

There are graphics that are often available for inclusion in reports or content media platforms as well as downloads for content analysis. I have included a few data visualization tools that (in addition to Excel) are useful in preparing data for analyses. This topic will be covered in the next chapter of the series.

Of particular interest for health policy content that was paramount in the expansion of the site or highlighting specific influencers of market access in cancer research is the History, Policy, and Laws link,

https://clinicaltrial.gov/ct2/about-site/history

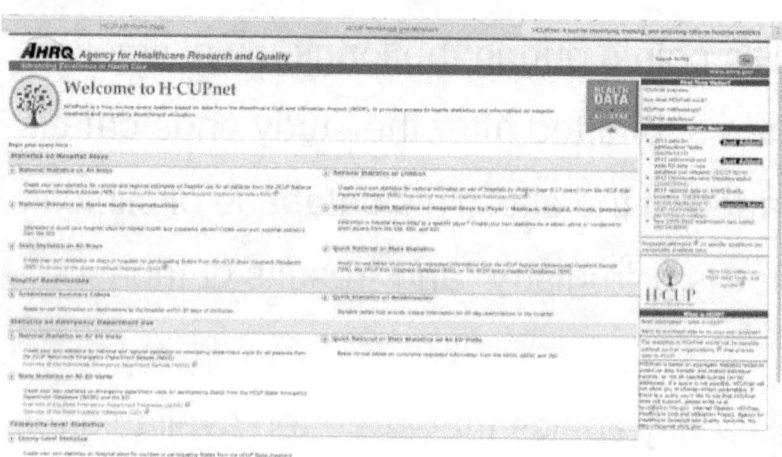

The Agency for Healthcare Research and Quality (AHRQ) hosts the HCUPnet, a free, on-line query system based on data from the Healthcare Cost and Utilization Project (HCUP). It provides access to health statistics and information on hospital inpatient and emergency department utilization and State Emergency Department Databases for ER visits that do not result in hospitalizations.

http://hcupnet.ahrq.gov

Data of Interest to Providers and Community

https://www.data.gov/health/

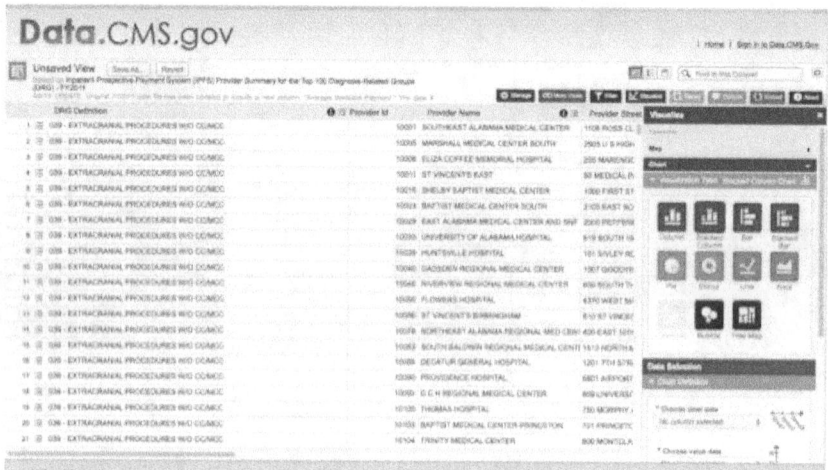

Data.gov links to over 245 state and federal healthcare datasets such as hospital charge data that can be searched by diagnosis-related groups (**DRG**)-- a system to classify hospital cases into specific groups, Agency for Healthcare Research and Quality (AHRQ), community healthcare centers, and Veterans Affairs data, for example. The screencast below lists a specific DRG and average and total payments for covered charges and Medicare payments. Visualization options are also listed in the expanded right column in addition options to export data for analyses, or filter by region for example.

The Surveillance, Epidemiology, and End Results (SEER) Program of the National Cancer Institute provides cancer statistics to help reduce the burden of cancer within the U.S. Released every spring with updated data from the prior November's submission date, the website currently includes 18 SEER registries from different years of diagnoses based on enrollment in the SEER program.

- (n) Fast Stats
  - State Cancer Profiles
  - Confidence Intervals for Ranks
  - Cancer Statistics Animator
  - Geographic Information System Portal
  - Prevalence and Cost of Care Projections
  - Cancer Query Systems

Tools
- Email
- Print Page
- Glossary

Interactive Tools

April 23, 2015: SEER cancer statistics through 2012 are now available.

The following Web-based systems provide access to statistical tables, graphs, and maps from various data sources.

Fast Stats
Build your own tables and graphs of key SEER and US cancer statistics.

State Cancer Profiles
Dynamic maps and graphs enabling the investigation of cancer trends at the county, state, and national levels.

Confidence Intervals for Ranks (CI*Rank)
Confidence intervals for ranks of age-adjusted US incidence and mortality rates by geographic region.

Cancer Statistics Animator
Animated graphs showing cancer trends over time.

NCI Geographic Information Systems (GIS) Portal
Interactive mapping and visualization of cancer related geo-spatial data.

Cancer Prevalence and Cost of Care Projections
Estimates and projects the national cost of cancer care through the year 2020.

Cancer Query Systems
Provides more flexibility and more cancer statistics than Fast Stats but requires more input from the user.

There are several interactive tools providing data access to answer a variety of health economics and clinical awareness questions. The ability to provide context for funding requests, awareness, or even brand positioning relies on a strong data informed narrative. A variety of linked data sources are available for review and analyses.

http://seer.cancer.gov/resources/

Data of Interest to Provider, Consumer, Community

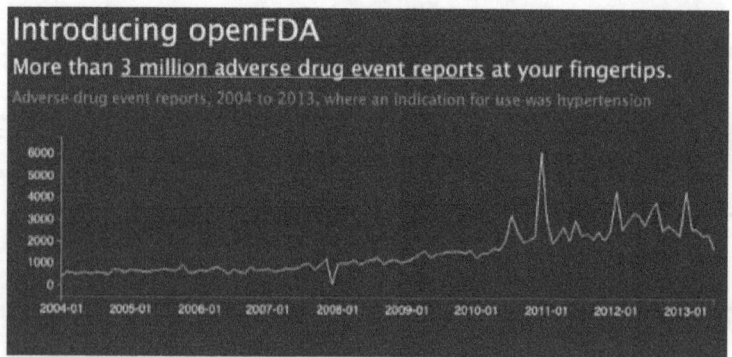

https://www.healthdata.gov

Healthdata.gov is a one-stop portal for free, publicly available data. Disease specific national and regional data is reported by CMS, Centers for Disease Control, Department of Health and Human Services in addition to state agencies, that cover over 1900 datasets.

Health Data Initiative Starter Kit provides an introduction overview to the types of data linked on the site.

I hope that you learned about a few new resources to help integrate data informed content for your medical communication objectives. Naturally the next step will be stepping through a few best practices to help prepare your data for analytics.

Stay tuned for the next chapter that will serve as a road map to help guide you through a few of the free options on the market. I feel that Excel is adequately covered elsewhere but I will likely include a few general concepts to help level-set our next discussion.

Next step will be creating the questions for the

narrative and visualizing the data…two options with free versions (with limited data security) are **Tableau Public** and **Plot.ly**
Have a look around and we can dive into the analytics and best practices for visualizing your data in the next chapter!

Tableau Public

Full disclosure, Tableau is my visualization tool of choice. It seems to be a little more intuitive to my non-IT brain although before you know it you might be writing code and finding new business opportunities for expanding your skills.

If you can manage simple excel tasks it shouldn't be too difficult to combine those skills and create, collaborate, share interactive charts and graphs, maps, live dashboards and then publish anywhere in your digital space.

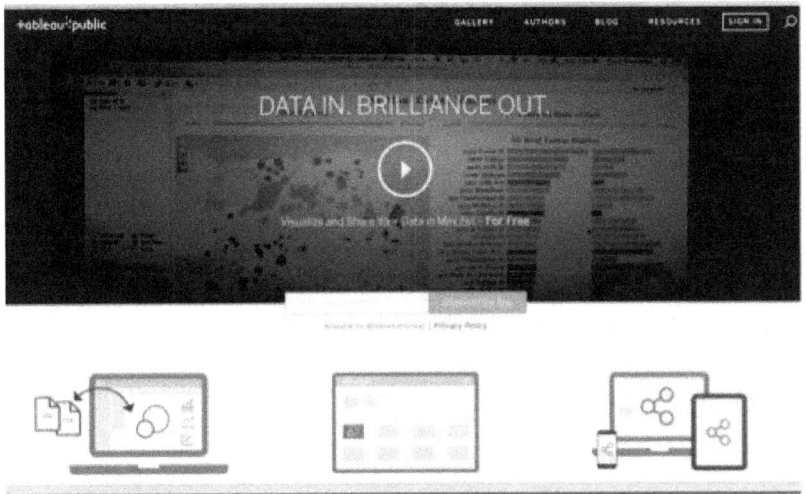

The next series will be asking a data question and using the data sources identified here to explore Tableau Public. Follow along at http://www.dataanddonuts.org for information about availability.

Plotl.y

Plotly is a tool with a free option powered for collaborative sharing. You have the ability to combine different data sources into a single visualization. Create charts for reports or dashboards and integrate into PowerPoint or email.

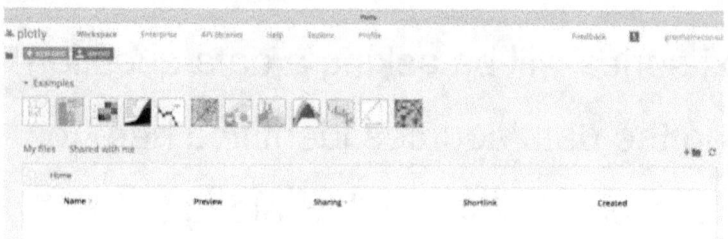

You may have noticed that a few government datasets allow integration with plotly at just a press of a button!

OpenRefine

Another free resource that evolved over the years was Google Refine. Now, no longer affiliated with Google, and renamed OpenRefine, it is a robust tool with a bit of a learning curve but strong community and online support tools. http://openrefine.org

The real sweet spot for OpenRefine is managing datasets that require cleaning before analysis.

A free, open source, powerful tool for working with messy data

Home

Download

Documentation

Community

Post archive

Mapping OpenRefine
Ecosystem

2014 survey results

A Governance Model for
OpenRefine

Using OpenRefine: a
manual

OpenRefine History

Tweets

Kerstin Forsberg in
Glasbox

Welcome!

OpenRefine (formerly Google Refine) is a powerful tool for working with messy data: cleaning it; transforming it from one format into another; extending it with web services; and linking it to databases like Freebase.

Please note that since October 2nd, 2012, Google is not actively supporting this project, which has now been rebranded to OpenRefine. Project development, documentation and promotion is now fully supported by volunteers. Find out more about the history of OpenRefine and how you can help the community.

Using OpenRefine - The Book

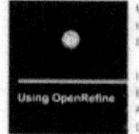

Using OpenRefine, by Ruben Verborgh and Max De Wilde, offers a great introduction to OpenRefine. Organized by recipes with hands-on examples, the book covers the following topics:

Import data in various formats

Explore datasets in a matter of seconds

Apply basic and advanced cell transformations

Deal with cells that contain multiple values

Create instantaneous links between datasets

6. Filter and partition your data easily with regular expressions

7. Use named-entity extraction on full-text fields to automatically identify topics

8. Perform advanced data operations with the General Refine Expression Language

Introduction to OpenRefine

Data freely available to the public

Public-Use Data Files and Documentation
http://www.cdc.gov/nchs/data_access/ftp_data.htm

"The National Center for Health Statistics (NCHS) is pleased to offer downloadable public-use data files through the Centers for Disease Control and Prevention's (CDC) FTP file server. Users of this service have access to data sets, documentation, and questionnaires from NCHS surveys and data collection systems. Downloading instructions are available in "readme" files.

Public-use data files are prepared and disseminated to provide access to the full scope of the data. This allows researchers to manipulate the data in a format appropriate for their analyses. NCHS makes every effort to release data collected through its surveys and data systems in a timely manner.

Users of NCHS public-use data files must comply with data use restrictions to ensure that the information will be used solely for statistical analysis or reporting purposes."

Datasets listed on the CDC website include:

National Health Care Surveys

- National Ambulatory Medical Care Survey (NAMCS)
- National Hospital Ambulatory Medical Care Survey (NHAMCS)
- National Hospital Discharge Survey (NHDS)
- National Survey of Ambulatory Surgery (NSAS)
- National Home and Hospice Care Survey (NHHCS)
- National Nursing Home Survey (NNHS)
- National Nursing Assistant Survey (NNAS)

National Vital Statistics Systems

- Vital Statistics Online - Access to downloadable datasets
- Natality (Births)
- Mortality (Deaths)
- Linked Birth/Infant Death
- Fetal Death
- National Mortality Followback Survey (NMFS)
- Matched Multiple Birth Data Set
- Mortality Component - Instruction Manuals
- MICAR Data Dictionary

National Health Interview Survey

- Questionnaires, Datasets, and Related Documentation

National Immunization Survey (NIS)

- Public-Use Data Files

Longitudinal Studies of Aging (LSOA)

- Data Files

Why data matters...

Let's use an example of determining the effectiveness of mammograms to detect breast cancer. Not to be too simplistic but lets consider how we might gather the necessary statistics. If we identify a positive mammogram what is the probability that we indeed detected cancer?

According to the American Cancer Society there are about 231,840 new cases of invasive breast cancer detected each year. Each year there are 38,770,390 mammographies performed. Since the accuracy of mammograms varies from 80% to 90% let's assume 90% for purposes of calculations. By adding the 10% of false positives to the estimated 231, 840 cases per year we have the probability of a positive mammogram indicating breast cancer to be 231,840/4108879 or roughly about 5%.

The cost of US mammograms vary from $100 with a reported average of $243 reported by a copay data aggregator, so those 38,770,390 mammograms cost about 3.8 billion dollars if we are using the low cost range.

Each case of breast cancer would cost about $18000 to diagnose and that does not even account for the biopsy required for confirmation which would likely double the 3.8 billion figure to above 7 billion yielding $34,000 dollars for the average cost of initial diagnosis.

One more step here. Since only one out of every 2000 women screened will have their life extended--if 38,770,390 women are screened each year that means that 19,385 women will have their lives extended by early screening to the cost of $361,103 per mammogram. This figure does not include treatment costs or other indirect costs related to the lives extended each year due to screenings.

Go find the data that is meaningful to you!

New data access...

I was invited to attend the National Health Statistics conference in Bethesda, Maryland. Here I discovered the Minnesota Population Center (MPC) and numerous datasets for exploring healthcare questions, demographics, and a variety of variables. You can search the site, http://www.ipums.org or find immediately relevant statistics here https://www.ihis.us/ihis-action/variables/group.

You will need a bit of trial and error to navigate through the website but if you are like me, a visual learner, within the hour you should have managed the learning curve enough to be functional.

I walked through the exhibition space and was able to collect reference material for my bookshelf. I was able to find free online sources for many of the same publications so you are in luck!

These resources are invaluable for creating context--a news story, proposal or need assessment, or disease state awareness.

Summary Health Statistics for the US Population: National Health Interview Survey, 2012

http://www.cdc.gov/nchs/data/series/sr_10/sr10_259.pdf

Healthy People 2010 Final Review: Progress Charts

http://www.cdc.gov/nchs/data/hpdata2010/hp2010_final_r eview.pdf

Health, United States, 2014 (special feature on adults aged 55 to 64)

http://www.cdc.gov/nchs/data/hus/hus14.pdf

###

Thank you for joining me on this data journey. If the information is helpful, won't you please take a moment to leave a review at your favorite retailer?

Thanks!

Bonny

Connect with me:

Twitter: http://twitter.com/graphemeconsult or http://twitter.com/dataanddonuts

Subscribe to my blog:

http://www.dataanddonuts.org

http://alzheimersdiseasethebrand.com

Improving Numeracy in Medicine

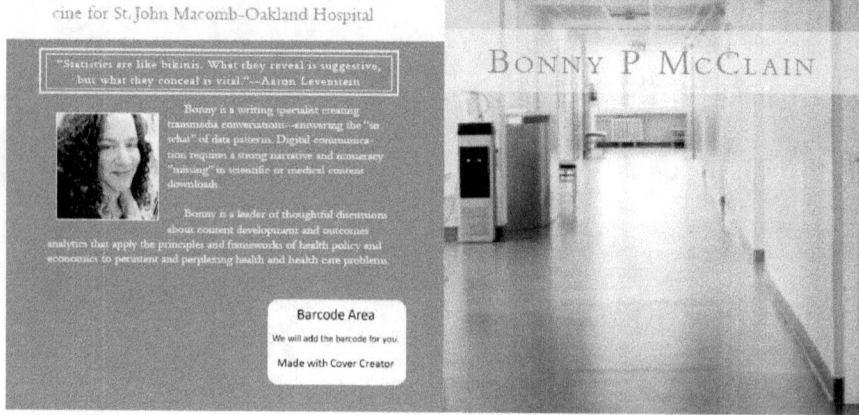

'This text is wonderfully written and clearly and concisely elucidates concepts critical for today's students, residents and practicing physicians. I'd recommend it for both undergraduate and graduate curriculum developers.'

Saroj Misra, DO, FACOFP, Director of Clinical Clerkship Curriculum for MSUCOM and Associate Program Director of Family Medicine for St. John Macomb-Oakland Hospital

"Statistics are like bikinis. What they reveal is suggestive, but what they conceal is vital."—Aaron Levenstein

Bonny is a writing specialist creating transmedia conversations—answering the "so what" of data patterns. Digital communication requires a strong narrative and numeracy "missing" in scientific or medical content downloads.

Bonny is a leader of thoughtful discussions about content development and outcomes analytics that apply the principles and frameworks of health policy and economics to persistent and perplexing health and health care problems.

Improving Numeracy in Medicine

BONNY P MCCLAIN

Barcode Area

We will add the barcode for you.

Made with Cover Creator

http://www.amazon.com/Bonny-P-McClain/e/B00J0M10OY/ref=sr_tc_2_0?qid=1450107924&sr=1-2-ent

www.ingramcontent.com/pod-product-compliance
Lightning Source LLC
Chambersburg PA
CBHW070924180526
45168CB00005B/2148